THE CURE FOR OBESITY:

Quick tips on how to overcome your

obsession with food and lose weight

BY

JAKE B. PETERS

TABLE OF CONTENTS

INTRODUCTION

Obesity has reached epidemic proportions in the United

States: more than 20% of adults are clinically obese as defined by a body mass index of 30 kg/m or higher, and an additional 30% are overweight. Environmental, behavioral, and genetic factors have been shown to contribute to the development of obesity. Elevated body mass index, particularly caused by abdominal or upper-body obesity, has been associated with several diseases and metabolic abnormalities, many of which have high morbidity and mortality. These include hyperinsulinemia, insulin resistance, type 2 diabetes, hypertension, dyslipidemia, coronary heart disease, gallbladder disease, and certain malignancies. This underscores the importance of identifying people at risk for obesity and its related disease states.

CHAPTER 1

WHAT CAUSE OBESITY

Obesity is a complex disease involving an excessive amount of body fat. Obesity isn't just a cosmetic concern. It's a medical problem that increases the risk of other diseases and health problems, such as heart disease, diabetes, high blood pressure, and certain cancers.

There are many reasons why some people have difficulty losing weight. Usually, obesity results from inherited, physiological and environmental factors, combined with diet, physical activity, and exercise choices.

The good news is that even modest weight loss can improve or prevent the health problems associated with obesity. A healthier diet increased physical activity, and behavior changes can help you lose weight. Prescription medications and weight-loss procedures are additional options for treating obesity.

Causes

Although there are genetic, behavioral, metabolic, and hormonal influences on body weight, obesity occurs when you take in more calories than you burn through normal daily activities and exercise. Your body stores these excess calories as fat.

In the United States, most people's diets are too high in calories — often from fast food and high-calorie beverages. People with obesity might eat more calories before feeling full, feel hungry sooner, or eat more due to stress or anxiety.

Many people who live in Western countries now have jobs that are much less physically demanding, so they don't tend to burn as many calories at work. Even daily activities use fewer calories, courtesy of conveniences such as remote controls, escalators, online shopping, and drive-through banks.

10 Leading Causes of Weight Gain and Obesity

Obesity is one of the biggest health problems in the world.

It's associated with several related conditions, collectively known as metabolic syndrome. These include

high blood pressure, elevated blood sugar, and a poor blood lipid profile.

People with metabolic syndrome are at a much higher risk of heart disease and type 2 diabetes, compared to those whose weight is in a normal range.

1. Genetics

Obesity has a strong genetic component. Children of parents with obesity are much more likely to have obesity than children of lean parents.

That doesn't mean that obesity is completely predetermined. What you eat can have a major effect on which genes are expressed and which are not.

Non-industrialized societies rapidly develop obesity when they start eating a typical Western diet. Their genes didn't change, but the environment and the signals they sent to their genes did.

Put simply, genetic components do affect your susceptibility to gaining weight. Studies on identical twins demonstrate this very well (2Trusted Source).

Summary

Some people appear to be genetically susceptible to weight gain and obesity.

2. Engineered Junk Foods

Heavily processed foods are often little more than refined ingredients mixed with additives.

These products are designed to be cheap, last long on the shelf, and taste so incredibly good that they are hard to resist.

By making foods as tasty as possible, food manufacturers are trying to increase sales. But they also promote overeating.

Most processed foods today don't resemble whole foods at all. These are highly engineered products, designed to get people hooked.

Summary

Stores are filled with processed foods that are hard to resist. These products also promote overeating.

3. Food Addiction

Many sugar-sweetened, high-fat junk foods stimulate the reward centers in your brain.

These foods are often compared to commonly abused drugs like alcohol, cocaine, nicotine, and cannabis.

Junk foods can cause addiction in susceptible individuals. These people lose control over their eating behavior, similar to people struggling with alcohol addiction losing control over their drinking behavior.

Addiction is a complex issue that can be very difficult to overcome. When you become addicted to something, you lose your freedom of choice and the biochemistry in your brain starts calling the shots for you.

Summary

Some people experience strong food cravings or addiction. This especially applies to sugar-sweetened, high-fat junk foods which stimulate the reward centers in the brain.

4. Aggressive Marketing

Junk food producers are very aggressive marketers.

Their tactics can get unethical at times and they sometimes try to market very unhealthy products as healthy foods.

These companies also make misleading claims. What's worse, they target their marketing specifically towards children.

In today's world, children are developing obesity and becoming diabetic and addicted to junk foods long before they're old enough to make informed decisions about these things.

Summary

Food producers spend a lot of money marketing junk food, sometimes specifically targeting children, who don't have the knowledge and experience to realize they are being misled.

5. Insulin

Insulin is a very important hormone that regulates energy storage, among other things.

One of its functions is to tell fat cells to store fat and to hold on to the fat they already carry.

The Western diet promotes insulin resistance in many overweight and individuals with obesity. This elevates insulin levels all over the body, causing energy to get stored in fat cells instead of being available for use.

While insulin's role in obesity is controversial, several studies suggest that high insulin levels have a causal role in the development of obesity.

One of the best ways to lower your insulin is to cut back on simple or refined carbohydrates while increasing fiber intake.

This usually leads to an automatic reduction in calorie intake and effortless weight loss — no calorie counting or portion control is needed.

Summary

High insulin levels and insulin resistance are linked to the development of obesity. To lower insulin levels, reduce your intake of refined carbs and eat more fiber.

6. Certain Medications

Many pharmaceutical drugs can cause weight gain as a side effect.

For example, antidepressants have been linked to modest weight gain over time.

Other examples include diabetes medication and antipsychotics.

These drugs don't decrease your willpower. They alter the function of your body and brain, reducing metabolic rate or increased appetite.

Summary

Some medications may promote weight gain by reducing the number of calories burned or increasing appetite.

7. Leptin Resistance

Leptin is another hormone that plays an important role in obesity.

It is produced by fat cells and its blood levels increase with higher fat mass. For this reason, leptin levels are especially high in people with obesity.

In healthy people, high leptin levels are linked to reduced appetite. When working properly, it should tell your brain how high your fat stores are.

The problem is that leptin isn't working as it should in many people who have obesity, because for some reason it cannot cross the blood-brain barrier (16Trusted Source).

This condition is called leptin resistance and is believed to be a leading factor in the pathogenesis of obesity.

Summary

Leptin, an appetite-reducing hormone, doesn't work in many individuals who have obesity.

8. Food Availability

Another factor that dramatically influences people's waist line is food availability, which has increased massively in the past few centuries.

Food, especially junk food, is everywhere now. Shops display tempting foods where they are most likely to gain your attention.

Another problem is that junk food is often cheaper than healthy, whole foods, especially in America.

Some people, especially in poorer neighborhoods, don't even have the option of purchasing real foods, like fresh fruit and vegetables.

Convenience stores in these areas only sell sodas, candy, and processed packaged junk foods.

How can it be a matter of choice if there is none?

Summary

In some areas, finding fresh, whole foods may be difficult or expensive, leaving people no choice but to buy unhealthy junk foods.

CHAPTER 2

THE CALORIE CONUNDRUM

Simply put, a calorie is a unit of energy. Calories indicate the energy content of the food and beverages you eat and drink. Understanding calories can help you make educated decisions about your diet and exercise.

There are three main sources of calories in the human diet. They come from the three macronutrients: carbohydrates, fat, and protein. Carbohydrates are the main source. They provide four calories per gram. Fat comes in second and offers more than twice as many calories, at nine calories per gram. Protein is the third source, which delivers four calories per gram. (Some countries use kilojoules instead of calories to measure food energy. This article uses calories. But here's the conversion rate you need—1 calorie = 4.2 kilojoules.)

A common question is whether all calories are created equal. On paper, it's hard to argue why they wouldn't be equal. Remember, calories are a measurement. So a calorie from fat should provide the same amount of energy as a calorie from protein. But really, this question should be posed to the gut.

Your gut absorbs almost all of the calories from the carbohydrates, protein, and fat you eat. But your gut treats fiber (a type of carbohydrate) differently than the other macronutrients. Instead of taking on all the calories, fiber has to offer, your gut will only absorb

about half. That's because fiber is difficult for the gut to digest completely.

On top of that, fiber easily absorbs water. This process can help you feel fuller for longer and helps you cut back how many calories you eat—or at least absorb. Combined with the other health benefits of fiber, it's no wonder that The American Heart Association recommends adults consume 25 grams per day.

DOES OVEREATING LEAD TO WEIGHT GAIN?

Overeating can lead to unwanted weight gain, and carrying excess weight can increase your cancer risk.

But it's not just about the unwanted calories. Overeating affects your body in a variety of ways.

So, what happens to your body when you overeat?

Overeating causes the stomach to expand beyond its normal size to adjust to a large amount of food. The expanded stomach pushes against other organs, making you uncomfortable. This discomfort can take the form of

feeling tired, sluggish, or drowsy. Your clothes may feel tight, too.

Eating too much food requires your organs to work harder. They secrete extra hormones and enzymes to break the food down.

To break down food, the stomach produces hydrochloric acid. If you overeat, this acid may back up into the esophagus resulting in heartburn. Consuming too much food that is high in fat, like pizza and cheeseburgers, may make you more susceptible to heartburn.

Your stomach may also produce gas, leaving you with an uncomfortable full feeling.

Your metabolism may speed up as it tries to burn off those extra calories. You may experience a temporary feeling of being hot, sweaty, or even dizzy.

Chapter3

The Hormonal mechanism of obesity

Hormones are chemical messengers that regulate processes in our bodies. They are one factor in causing

Obesity . The hormones leptin and insulin, sex hormones, and growth hormone influence our appetite, metabolism (the rate at which our body burns kilojoules for energy), and body fat distribution. People who are obese have levels of these hormones that encourage abnormal metabolism and the accumulation of body fat.

A system of glands, known as the endocrine system, secretes hormones into our bloodstream. The endocrine system works with the nervous system and the immune system to help our body cope with different events and stresses. Excesses or deficits of hormones can lead to obesity and, on the other hand, obesity can lead to changes in hormones.

Obesity and leptin

The hormone leptin is produced by fat cells and is secreted into our bloodstream. Leptin reduces a person's appetite by acting on specific centers of their brain to reduce their urge to eat. It also seems to control how the body manages its store of body fat.

Because leptin is produced by fat, leptin levels tend to be higher in people who are obese than in people of normal weight. However, despite having higher levels of this

appetite-reducing hormone, people who are obese aren't as sensitive to the effects of leptin and, as a result, tend not to feel full during and after a meal. Ongoing research is looking at why leptin messages aren't getting through to the brain in people who are obese.

Obesity and insulin

Insulin, a hormone produced by the pancreas, is important for the regulation of carbohydrates and the metabolism of fat. Insulin stimulates glucose (sugar) uptake from the blood in tissues such as muscles, the liver, and fat. This is an important process to make sure that energy is available for everyday functioning and to maintain normal levels of circulating glucose.

In a person who is obese, insulin signals are sometimes lost and tissues are no longer able to control glucose levels. This can lead to the development of type II diabetes and metabolic syndrome.

Obesity and sex hormones

Body fat distribution plays an important role in the development of obesity-related conditions such as heart disease, stroke, and some forms of arthritis. Fat around

our abdomen is a higher risk factor for disease than fat stored on our bottom, hips, and thighs. It seems that estrogens and androgens help to decide body fat distribution. Estrogens are sex hormones made by the ovaries in pre-menopausal women. They are responsible for prompting ovulation every menstrual cycle.

Men and postmenopausal women do not produce much estrogen in their testes (testicles) or ovaries. Instead, most of their estrogen is produced in their body fat, although at much lower amounts than what is produced in pre-menopausal ovaries. In younger men, androgens are produced at high levels in the testes. As a man gets older, these levels gradually decrease.

The changes with age in the sex hormone levels of both men and women are associated with changes in body fat distribution. While women of childbearing age tend to store fat in their lower body ('pear-shaped'), older men and postmenopausal women tend to increase the storage of fat around their abdomen ('apple-shaped'). Postmenopausal women who are taking estrogen supplements don't accumulate fat around their

abdomen. Animal studies have also shown that a lack of estrogen leads to excessive weight gain.

Obesity and growth hormone

The pituitary gland in our brain produces growth hormone, which influences a person's height and helps build bone and muscle. Growth hormone also affects metabolism (the rate at which we burn kilojoules for energy). Researchers have found that growth hormone levels in people who are obese are lower than in people of normal weight.

Inflammatory factors and obesity

Obesity is also associated with low-grade chronic inflammation within the fat tissue. Excessive fat storage leads to stress reactions within fat cells, which in turn leads to the release of pro-inflammatory factors from the fat cells themselves and immune cells within the adipose (fat) tissue.

Obesity hormones as a risk factor for disease

Obesity is associated with an increased risk of several diseases, including cardiovascular disease, stroke, and

several types of cancer, and with decreased longevity (shorter life span) and lower quality of life. For example, the increased production of estrogen in the fat of older women who are obese is associated with an increase in breast cancer risk, indicating that the source of estrogen production is important.

Behavior and obesity hormones

People who are obese have hormone levels that encourage the accumulation of body fat. It seems that behaviors such as overeating and lack of regular exercise, over time, 'reset' the processes that regulate appetite and body fat distribution to make the person physiologically more likely to gain weight. The body is

always trying to maintain balance, so it resists any short-term disruptions such as crash dieting.

Various studies have shown that a person's blood leptin level drops after a low-kilojoule diet. Lower leptin levels may increase a person's appetite and slow down their metabolism. This may help to explain why crash dieters

usually regain their lost weight. Leptin therapy may one day help dieters to maintain their weight loss in the long term, but more research is needed before this becomes a reality.

There is evidence to suggest that long-term behavior changes, such as healthy eating and regular exercise, can re-train the body to shed excess body fat and keep it off. Studies have also shown that weight loss as a result of a healthy diet and exercise or bariatric surgery leads to improved insulin resistance, decreased inflammation, and beneficial modulation of obesity hormones. Weight loss is also associated with a decreased risk of developing heart disease, stroke, type II diabetes, and some cancers.

Chapter 4

How sugar drives obesity and fat gain around the stomach

Many dietary and lifestyle habits can lead to weight gain and cause you to put on excess body fat.

Consuming a diet high in added sugars, such as those found in sweetened beverages, candy, baked goods, and sugary cereals, is a contributing factor in weight gain and chronic health conditions, including obesity, heart disease, and diabetes.

How added sugar intake leads to weight gain and increased body fat is complex and involves many factors.

Here are 6 reasons why added sugar is fattening.

1. High in empty calories

Added sugars are sweeteners added to foods and beverages to improve the taste. Some common types include fructose, corn syrup, cane sugar, and agave.

Excess sugar may cause you to pack on weight because it's high in calories while offering few other nutrients.

For example, 2 tablespoons (30 ml) of the common sweetener corn syrup contain 120 calories — exclusively from carbs.

Added sugars are often referred to as empty calories, as they're relatively high in calories yet void of nutrients like vitamins, minerals, protein, fat, and fiber, which your body needs to function optimally.

Plus, foods and beverages that typically contain a lot of added sugars, such as ice cream, candy, soda, and cookies, tend to be loaded with calories as well.

Though using small amounts of added sugar is unlikely to cause weight gain, regularly indulging in foods high in added sugars may cause you to gain excess body fat quicker and more drastically.

SUMMARY

Added sugar is a source of empty calories and offers little in terms of nutrition. Foods rich in added sugars tend to be high in calories, which can cause weight gain.

2. Impacts blood sugar and hormone levels

It's well known that eating sugary foods significantly raises your blood sugar levels.

Though enjoying sweet food infrequently isn't likely to harm health, daily consumption of large amounts of added sugar can lead to chronically elevated blood sugar levels.

Prolonged elevated blood sugar — known as hyperglycemia — can cause serious harm to your body, including weight gain.

One way hyperglycemia leads to weight gain is by promoting insulin resistance.

Insulin is a hormone produced by your pancreas that moves sugar from your blood into cells, where it can be used for energy. Insulin is also involved in energy storage, telling your cells when to store energy as either fat or glycogen, the storage form of glucose.

Insulin resistance is when your cells stop responding properly to insulin, which leads to elevated sugar and insulin levels.

High blood sugar levels impair normal cell function and promote inflammation, which increases insulin resistance, furthering this destructive cycle.

Though cells become resistant to insulin's effect on blood sugar uptake, they remain responsive to the hormone's role in fat storage, meaning that fat storage is increased.

This phenomenon is known as selective insulin resistance.

This is why insulin resistance and high blood sugar are associated with increased body fat — specifically in the belly area.

Additionally, high blood sugar levels and insulin resistance interfere with leptin, a hormone that plays a major role in energy regulation — including calorie intake and burning — and fat storage. Leptin decreases the hunger and helps reduce food intake.

Likewise, high-sugar diets are associated with leptin resistance, which increases appetite and contributes to weight gain and excess body fat (13Trusted Source).

SUMMARY

High-sugar diets contribute to prolonged elevated blood sugar, insulin resistance, and leptin resistance — all of which are linked to weight gain and excess body fat.

3. Foods high in added sugar tend to be less filling

Foods and beverages that are packed with added sugar, such as cakes, cookies, ice cream, candy, and soda, tend to be low in or completely lacking in protein, a nutrient essential for blood sugar control that promotes feelings of fullness.

Protein is the most filling macronutrient. It does this by slowing digestion, keeping blood sugar levels stable, and regulating hunger hormones.

For example, protein helps reduce levels of ghrelin, a hormone that drives appetite and increases calorie intake.

Conversely, eating protein stimulates the production of peptide YY (PYY) and glucagon-like peptide 1 (GLP-1), hormones associated with feelings of fullness that help reduce food intake.

Eating foods rich in carbs — particularly refined carbs high in added sugars — yet low in protein can negatively impact fullness and may lead to weight gain by causing you to eat more at subsequent meals throughout the day.

High-sugar foods also tend to be low in fiber, a nutrient that can increase feelings of fullness and reduce appetite — though not as much as protein.

SUMMARY

High-sugar foods and beverages are generally low in protein and fiber, nutrients that are essential for keeping you feeling full and satisfied.

4. Displace healthy foods

If most of your diet revolves around foods high in added sugars, chances are you're missing out on important nutrients.

Protein, healthy fats, fiber, vitamins, and minerals are all nutrients found in whole, nutritious foods that your body needs to function optimally and stay healthy. They're usually lacking in sugary products.

Additionally, refined foods and beverages that are high in added sugar don't have beneficial compounds like antioxidants, which are concentrated in foods like olive oil, nuts, beans, egg yolks, and brightly colored vegetables and fruits.

Antioxidants help protect your cells from damage caused by highly reactive molecules called free radicals.

Oxidative stress — an imbalance between antioxidants and free radicals — has been linked to a variety of chronic conditions, such as heart disease and certain cancers.

Unsurprisingly, diets high in added sugars increase your risk of the same chronic diseases linked to oxidative stress, as well as your risk of obesity and weight gain.

Eating foods high in added sugar displaces nutrient-rich, healthy foods like vegetables, fruits, proteins, and healthy fats — which could negatively impact your weight and overall health.

SUMMARY

Added sugars displace healthy foods, may lead to weight gain, and increase your risk of chronic health conditions like heart disease.

5. May cause you to overeat

Eating too much added sugar — particularly foods rich in a type of sugar called fructose — can significantly increase levels of the hunger-promoting hormone ghrelin while decreasing levels of the appetite-suppressing hormone peptide YY.

Fructose may also increase appetite by affecting a part of your brain called the hypothalamus. The hypothalamus is responsible for many functions, including appetite regulation, calories burned, as well as carb and fat metabolism.

Animal studies indicate that fructose impacts signaling systems in your hypothalamus, increasing levels of hunger-stimulating neuropeptides — molecules that communicate with one another, influencing brain activity — while decreasing fullness signals.

What's more, your body is predisposed to crave sweetness. Research shows that sugar consumption is driven by the pleasure derived from the sweet taste of sugary drinks and foods.

Studies suggest that sweet-tasting foods activate certain parts of your brain that are responsible for pleasure and reward, which may enhance your craving for sweet food.

Additionally, sugar may increase your desire for highly palatable, calorie-rich foods.

A study in 19 people found that consuming 10 ounces (300 ml) of a sugary drink led to an increased response to pictures of high-calorie, palatable foods like cookies and pizza and reduced levels of the appetite-suppressing hormone GLP-1, compared to a placebo.

Thus, the impact of sugar on hormones and brain activity may increase your desire for sweet-tasting foods and may encourage overeating — which can lead to weight gain.

SUMMARY

Sugar affects appetite-regulating hormones and reward centers in your brain, which may increase the desire for highly palatable foods and cause you to overeat.

6. Linked to obesity and chronic disease

Numerous studies have linked high intake of added sugars to weight gain and chronic conditions, such as obesity, heart disease, and diabetes.

This effect has been seen in both adults and children.

A recent review of 30 studies on more than 242,000 adults and children found a significant association between sugar-sweetened beverages and obesity.

Countless studies link sugary foods and beverages to weight gain in different populations, including pregnant women and teens.

Another study on 6,929 children demonstrated that those between the ages of 6 and 10 who consumed more added sugars had significantly more body fat than children who consumed less added sugar.

Studies show that diets high in added sugar can increase your risk of chronic health conditions as well.

In a population study of more than 85,000 people, the risk of dying from heart disease was more than twice as high in those consuming 25% or more of their daily

calories from added sugars, compared to those who consumed less than 10% of calories from added sugar.

What's more, added sugar is strongly associated with an increase in heart disease in children through its role in raising body fat, cholesterol, and triglyceride levels — all significant risk factors for heart disease.

Sugar-sweetened beverages are also associated with the development of type 2 diabetes in adults.

Plus, added sugar consumption may increase your risk of depression, a condition that may promote weight gain.

SUMMARY

Consuming too much-added sugar can cause weight gain and significantly increase your risk of chronic conditions like obesity, heart disease, and diabetes.

CHAPTER 5

THE OBESITY-FIX DIET

The obesity epidemic has no single or simple solution. It's a complex problem that requires a multifaceted approach. Policymakers; state and local organizations; business, school, and community leaders; childcare and healthcare professionals; and individuals must work together to create an environment that supports healthy lifestyles.

State and Local Programs

Resources are available to help disseminate consistent public health recommendations and evidence-based practices for state, local, territorial, and tribal public health organizations, grantees, and practitioners.

Community Efforts

To reverse the obesity epidemic, community efforts should focus on supporting healthy eating and active living in a variety of settings. Learn about different

efforts that can be used in early childhood care, hospitals, schools, and food service venues.

Healthy Living

The key to achieving and maintaining a healthy weight isn't short-term dietary changes; it's about a lifestyle that includes healthy eating and regular physical activity.

Assessing Your Weight

Body mass index (BMI) and waist circumference as screening tools to estimate weight status and potential disease risk.

Healthy Weight

Achieving and maintaining a healthy weight with healthy eating, physical activity, optimal sleep, and stress reduction.

MyPlate Planexternal icon

Personalized plan suggesting what and how much to eat from each food group to meet your calorie needs.

Physical Activity Basics

Benefits of physical activity and the recommended amounts of weekly physical activity for various groups.

www.ingramcontent.com/pod-product-compliance
Lightning Source LLC
LaVergne TN
LVHW052103160826
845678LV00015B/3328

* 9 7 9 8 3 5 3 1 8 5 7 8 9 *